A Hospital Humor Book

Food for Thought ...In The Bed!

R. Neil Laughlin

Don't Read Another Page
Until You've Read This One!

Here's how to get the most
enjoyment out of this book.

1) Pick a saying, any saying, and read
   it as it is written. THEN...

2) read it again, adding the words
   "in the bed" at the end.

The result will either be

a) very, very funny, or

b) a deeper the meaning of the
   original saying.

EITHER WAY, you will find a
treasure of truths that will bring
you hours of enjoyment.

DEDICATION

Food For Thought...In The Bed is dedicated to the doctors, the physician assistants, the nurses and all the other support staffs of Central Maine Cardio Vascular Institute in Lewiston, ME, a part of Central Maine Medical .

A no more competent medical team exists ... anywhere in this country, not in Boston, not in Cleveland, not in, well you get my point. Not Anywhere!

Their secret, aside from being top-notch trained individuals, is that from the top to the bottom, they treat each patient - and the patient's family - as people. They are truly caring caregivers!

Thank you all for all you did for me... and my family. You're the BEST!

SPECIAL THANKS
To Paul Karwowski who's help with
the cover design was invaluable.

1,001 Bites
of food for thought

1. The wise man is the one who makes you think he is dumb.

2. Nothing is lost until your mother can't find it.

3. Shallow thinking people can easily drown in small puddles of intelligence.

4. Courtesy costs nothing.

5. Actions cannot be rewritten.

6. Proper preparation can be a life saving exercise.

7. Courtesy cost nothing, but can return great rewards.

8. Except one-legged man everyone
   puts pants on
   one leg at a time.

9. What you can not touch is more
   valuable than what you can touch.

10. Your mood is one of only a few
    things you can control.

11. Sometimes you have to step back
    to move forward.

12. Failure is only failure when you
    stop trying to succeed.

13. Following the path of others
    results in limited views.

14. A person is never too old
    to learn.

15. What is H20? Caring. Two parts
    hug and one part open-mind.

16. Silent company often heals more than worlds of advice.

17. We are spiritual beings going through a temporary human experience.

18. Common sense is instinct. Enough of it is genius.

19. Adventure can be real happiness. No man is without enemies.

20. Good health is a man's best wealth.

21. As you slide down the banister of life, may the splinters never point your direction.

22. Nothing dared, nothing gained.

23.   Punctuality is the expression of commitment.

24.   The greater one's guilt, the greater the need to place blame elsewhere.

25.   You must be willing to act today in order to succeed.

26.   Understand yourself so you may understand others.

27.   There is no fear for the one whose thoughts is not confused.

28.   We secure our friends not by accepting favors but by doing them.

29.   Love is a present that can be given every single day of your live.

30. No man ever yet became great by imitation.

31. The one thing contained in everything is Wisdom.

32. It is what it is, until you chose to change it.

33. Narrow thinking people live on window ledges.

34. Arrogance is usually spawned from ignorance.

35. Living in the Past negates an opportunity to build a better future.

36. When the moment comes, take the last one.

37. The nicest place to be is in someone's happy thoughts.

38. Necessity does everything well.

39. A new friend helps you break out of an old routine.

40. A danger foreseen is half avoided.

41. A diversity of friends is a credit to your flexible nature.

42. A gathering of friends brings lots of luck this evening.

43. Dare to dream, hope, believe, and love. Not to do this is to live a boring life.

44. A good laugh and a good cry both cleanse the mind.

45. What is a friend! A single soul dwelling is two bodies.

46. You will stumble into the happiness of your life.

47. This is a good time to consider formally helping others.

48. A great pleasure in life is doing what others say you can't.

49. A journey of a thousand miles begins with one small step.

50. You aspire to great things? Begin with little ones.

51. Cast your hook in the pool where you least expect it. There will be the fish.

52. A smile can always overcome the barrier of language.

53. Music is the champagne that fills the empty glass of silence.

54. You will enjoy good health; you will be surrounded by luxury.

55. You will travel far and wide, both for pleasure and business.

56. Good people are good because they've
come to wisdom through failure.

57. Your deeds speak so much louder than another's words.

58. Your love light shines on another.
59. Instead of giving someone a piece of your mind, give them the peace of your mind.

60. Dealing with tangled Christmas lights, tells lot about the person.

61. Poetry produces preponderance.

62. Confidence and Ignorance can produce short-term success.

63. A poem is the essence of truth distilled from an ocean of babble.

64. To succeed, you have to be seen for who you are.

65. Rank has its privilege…and its odor.

66. To know your limits is to try to go beyond them.

67. Awards are milestones, not millstones in life.

68.   Smile and rejoice, fortune is
        smiling on you.

69.   The true merit of your actions will
        be measured by
         how others perceive them.

70.   The seeking of Perfection focuses
        on process; success on results.

71.   Knowledge equips you to filter the
        view of others.

72.   Playing second position is
        imitation;
         playing first position is initiation.

73.   You must find the harmony
        in our world of conflicting spheres.

74.   Eventually everyone dies, but not
        everyone lives.

75. The "self-pity" song is best sung in the shower.

76. Speaking badly of your significant other brings your own judgment into question.

77. A great man never ignores the simplicity of a child.

78. Your character can be described as natural and unrestrained.

79. You will find luck when you go home.

80. Write injuries in dust, benefits in marble.

81. A new voyage will fill your life with untold memories.

82. A fine is a tax for doing wrong. A tax is a fine for doing well.

83. Most Success springs from an obstacle or failure.

84. Your dreams are expressions from the book of your soul.

85. Your aspirations are met with success soon.

86. You will finally solve a difficult problem that means much to you.

87. You will inherit some money or a small piece of land.

88. Prosperity is a way of living and thinking, and not just having money or material things.

89. People make plans; fate makes the plan successful.

90. The situation is changeable, yet you cannot push the river.

91. Never argue with a fool.
92. May life throw you a pleasant curve.

93. Don't let the status quo stand in the way of a good idea.

94. Victory and defeat are transitory,
their longevity determined by your
will.

95. Greed may be good for an
individual,
but not necessarily one's for
society.

96. Ultimately the material is
immaterial.

97. What and How without Why
usually results in
miscommunication and failure of
your goal.

98. Those who say they have all the
answers, don't.

99. One look is worth ten thousand
words.

100.　Tolerance of others' thoughts is key to a long-term relationship.

101.　To have "class" does not require merely
having "cash".

102.　Smothering is NOT mothering…nor is it fathering.

103.　We are all terminal at some time and point. We just don't know our expiration date.

104.　A poor person can live a richer life than a wealthy person.

105.　Why do people who "speak from the heart" read from a prepared text?

106.　Peace of mind is more valuable than a "piece of money".

107. Don't be afraid to take a chance when the opportunity of a lifetime presents itself.

108. In order remain young, on must change.

109. Don't play for safety – it's the most dangerous thing in the world.

110. Good news of a long-awaited event will arrive soon.

111. Rivers need springs.

112. It is much wiser to take advice than to give it.

113. The universe will reward you for taking risks on its behalf.

114. He who knows others is wise. He who knows himself is enlightened.

115. In a gentle way, you can shake the world.

116. He who believes is strong. He who doubts is weak.

117. Look ahead or you won't get ahead.

118. Our deeds determine us, as much as we determine our deeds.

119. As long as you are alive, you have a chance to succeed.

120. Quantity often times dilutes Quality.

121. Today's enemy may be

tomorrow's ally

122. A moment of understanding can eliminate years of remorse.

123. Failure is as great a teacher as knowledge.

124. Mistakes are learning opportunities.

125. Most people are about as happy as they make up their minds to be.

126. There is no substitute for good manners, except,
     maybe fast reflexes.

127. People have great respect for you.

128. Listening well is as essential to all true conversation as talking well.

129. Bend the rod while still hot.

130. No problem can stand the assault
of sustained thinking.

131. Someone can read your mind.

132. The challenged life is your best
therapist.

133. Perceived failure is oftentimes
success
   trying to be born in
   a bigger way.

134. No man is without enemies.

135. Your true wisdom manifests itself
in your instincts.

136. Only a life lived for others is a life
worthwhile.

137. Little and often makes much.

138. Even the smartest person can learn something from the dumbest.

139. Perpetual optimism is a force multiplier.

140. People are just as happy
    as they make up
    their minds to be.

141. Pure love is to give without a thought of receiving anything in return.

142. Desire, like the atom, is explosive with creative force.

143. Pursue your work with all due seriousness.

144. Listen to yourself more often.

145.   The loss of which is unknown is
       no loss at all.

146.   Resting on ones laurels can result
       in a prickly situation.

147.   Today, your success depends upon
       working with people of all
       different beliefs, nationality and
       color.

148.   Life will love you back as much as
       you love it.

149.   Respect for others is peace.
       Respect for yourself is happiness.

150.   The ultimate journey is going
       inside oneself.

151.   It takes courage to lead a life; any
       life.

152. It is more difficult to judge yourself
     than to judge others.

153. Ride your ambition
     to the skies.

154. We can't control the wind, but we can always
     adjust the sails.

155. Nobody ever drowned in his own sweat.

156. Everything you do, do to make
     your heart sing.

157. Don't expect romantic attachments
     to be strictly logical or rational.

158. Read a novel – and learn more
     about life.

159. The smart thing is to prepare for the unexpected.

160. Plan for the best, prepare for the worst.

161. Experience is what you harvest when you don't reap what you wanted.

162. When everyday becomes routine, it's time to get a new every day.

163. Today brings out the performer in you.

164. You must be able to face yourself before you can truly face the world.

165. Education and intelligence are not the same thing!

166. Confidence isn't something that you get. It's something that you are.

167. Good character is more to be praised than outstanding talent.

168. Home is where the heart is.

169. You'll never find a better sparring partner than adversity.

170. Depend on your feet; you can climb the highest mountain.

171. Chance favors those in motion.

172. Everyone around you is rooting for you.
Don't give up!

173. Bumps in the road are part of your life's journey.

174. Do not wish to be anything but what you are, and try to be that perfectly.

175. Don't let ambitions overshadow small success.

176. If you want people to like you, like yourself first.

177. He who knows others is wise. He who knows himself is enlightened.

178. Example is better than perception.

179. Courtesy is the password to safety.

180. Don't fret. All your friends will be able to zig whenever you zag.

181. You will find yourself in a position of dignity in the end.

182. Doing best this moment puts you in the best place for the next moment.

183. Burnt bridges are hard to cross.

184. Conquer the "devil within" before trying to conquer the devil outside.

185. Education is not filling a bucket but lighting a fire.

186. May the warm winds of heaven blow softly upon your spirit.

187. Today's virtue may be tomorrow's vice and vice versa.

188. There is a time to be practical – NOW!

189. Taking no risk could be taking the greatest risk.

190. Enlightenment begets Guilt, while Guilt mothers regret.

191. Your core values will be the ink of your autobiography.

192. Visualize to Materialize. If you can't see it you can't do or be it.

193. Nothing lasts forever and most things don't last very long.

194. Success or Failure is one step over the line between   Brilliance and Stupidity.

195. The person who learns to laugh at himself will never cease to be amused.

196. There is no wisdom greater than kindness.

197. Temptation resistant is the true measure of character.

198. Well begun is only half done.

199. This is really a lovely day. Congratulations!

200. Take a vacation. You will have unexpected gains.

201. To be sure you hit the target, shoot first and call what you hit the target.

202. If absolute can be defined, then absolute is not absolute anymore.

203. Impossible standards just make life difficult.

204. If you never change your mind, why have one?

205. Good Luck is a hop, skip and a jump away. Hop to it!

206. The Truth hurts when viewed from a false reality.

207. Only a tradition of innovation can last... business and personal.

208. One that would have the fruit must climb the tree.

209. A cheerful letter or message is on its way to you.

210. Two eyes, two ears, one mouth: use in proportion.

211. You are more likely to give than to give in.

212. Today means action. Carry out your plan.

213. If you want to be a "Big Fish" don't swim in a small pond.

214. This is your day! Expect great results with those ongoing works.

215. You are about to become $8.95 poorer. ($7.95 plus tax if you had the buffet.)

216. Water not only can keep a ship afloat, it also can sink it.

217. Fool yourself, rob yourself; know yourself and win the world.

218.   Differed maintenance turns
          mole hills into mountains.

219.   Nothing is wrong with visiting the
          Past;
          just don't make it your home.

220.   People try things, because they
          just don't want it enough.

221.   You don't get in life what you
          want; you get in life
           what you are.

222.   Opportunity always knocks at the
          least opportune moment.

223.   Turn on the charm. You'll be
           glad you did.

224.   Where there is no vision,
           the people perish.

225. Pay attention, an opportunity will knock on your door.

226. You cannot become rich except by enriching others.

227. Thinking is heavily endorsed.

228. You need to live authentically, and you can't ignore that.

229. No one can make you feel inferior without your consent.

230. You would remember that Good Samaritan, if he only had good intentions.

231. Some people dream of accomplishments; others stay awake and do them.

232. When you awaken tomorrow,
     solutions to your problems will be
     clear.

233. Tradition can be a deterrent to
     innovation and progress.

234. Dedication to duty is more
     important
     than duty to dedication.

235. Winning at all costs is ultimately
     losing.

236. The specter casted by Fear is
     always
      greater than Fear itself.

237. An inflexible mind obstructs
     one's ability to have a full view.

238. It is not the length of time one
lives, but what
  one does with it that truly matters.

239. Over optimism is usually Greed in
sheep's clothing.

240. Everything cannot be exciting,
otherwise you would not know
what is exciting.

241. Life is a labyrinth, so you better
develop a map.

242. A wise person praises others in
public and criticizes in private.

243. The best thing about growing older
is that it takes such a long time.

244. Your happiness is around the next
corner, wealth down the street.

245. You are the only flower of
meditation in the wilderness.

246. Life's a continual negotiation.

247. Reality depends upon who is most
persuasive.

248. Courtesy is cumbersome to them
that know it not.

249. People who claim not to have any
vices, usually don't have
much virtue either.

250. Getting the right answers is only
possible when you ask the right
questions.

251. Good things will come to you in
due course of time.

252. The truth always shines
through…eventually.

253. Happy news is on its way.

254. Happiness is a state of mind.

255. Fear can keep us up all night long,
but faith makes one fine pillow.

256. Happiness is not a reward, it's a
consequence.

257. If the table moves,
move with it.

258. Greet the world every morning
with curiosity
and hope.

259. For everything there is a season.

260. The road to success is always under construction.

261. Catch on fire with enthusiasm and people will come for miles to watch you burn.

262. He who is afraid of asking is ashamed of learning.

263. Happiness is not found in having what you want but rather in wanting what you have.

264. Somewhere, deep inside, we all can fly.

265. A short saying oft contains much wisdom.

266. Dream lofty dreams, and as you dream, so shall you become.

267. Leaders are readers.

268. Don't scrap everything!
See what you can salvage.

269. A charming friendship is in the
making.

270. You can see through people or,
you can see people through.

271. You're a practical person with
your feet on the ground.

272. You could prosper in the field of
medical research.

273. Versatility is one of your
outstanding traits.

274. Good news will be brought to you
by mail.

275. You love sports, horses and
     Gambling…but not to excess.

276. Your love life will be happy and
     harmonious.

277. You are kind-hearted and
     hospitable,
      cheerful and well-liked.

278. You have a deep interest in all that
     is artistic.

279. You will spend old age in comfort
     and material wealth.

280. You have an ability to sense
      and know higher truth.

281. A good time to finish up old tasks.

282. You are very expressive and
     positive

in word, act, and feeling.

283. Your emotional nature is strong
      and sensitive.

284. The two hardest things to handle in
      life
        are failure an success.

285. Peace begins with a smile.

286. One of the best ways to persuade
      others
        is with your ears – listen.

287. You grow up the first day you
      have a good laugh at yourself.

288. Pessimism never won any battles.

289. Put the data you have uncovered to
      a beneficial use.

290. There will be plenty of time to work hard; enjoy yourself!

291. As soon as you feel too old to do a thing, do it.

292. We are taught by every person we meet.

293. Pay attention, an opportunity will knock on your door.

294. The fish who keeps his mouth closed doesn't get hooked.

295. Your cheerful outlook is one of your assets.

296. Avoid taking unnecessary gambles.

297. Your cell phone is making you a prisoner of yourself.

298.   A cloud is an inspiration,
          bringing it to ground takes time.

299.   Avoid compulsively making things
          worse.

300.   At the end of the day, think "what
          has this day brought me?" and then
          ask, "What have I given it?"

301.   There can be no existence of evil
          as a force to the healthy-minded
          individual.

302.   No man is free who is not master
          of himself.

303.   Soon life will become
          more interesting.

304.   Enjoy what you have! Never mind
          fame and power.

305. Minor aches today are likely to pay off handsomely tomorrow.

306. Reading to the mind is what exercise is to the body.

307. It's fun being a kid.

308. Flying is simple. Not hitting the ground is hard.

309. Nothing in the world is accomplished without passion.

310. Great acts of kindness will befall you in the coming months.

311. Nothing ventured, nothing gained.

312. The greatest pleasure in life is doing what people say you cannot do.

313. Seek to assert your devotion when a worthy situation arises.

314. Punctuality is the expression of commitment.

315. The first man gets the oyster, the second man gets the shell.

316. Live each day well and wisely.

317. A secret is best kept by one.

318. People are apt to settle a question rightly when it is discussed freely.

319. This Moment real. The Past memory. The Future Hope. Only the Present is real.

320. Remember to order your take out also?

321. Learn from how people in the arts react to criticism.

322. The face is the roadmap to a person's feelings.

323. People don't care how much you know until they know how much you care.

324. Never compare yourself to the best others can do, instead compare yourself to the best you can do.

325. Kiss is not a kiss without the heart.

326. Search your own heart with diligence for out of it flows the issues of life.

327. Minds are like parachutes. The only function when they are open.

328. If we do not change our direction, we are likely to end up where we intended to be.

329. Patience makes lighter what Sorrow may not heal.

330. He that gives should not remember; He that receives should never forget.

331. Enthusiasm is contagious. Not having enthusiasm is also contagious.

332. Do your work with your whole heart and you will succeed.

333. Minutes are worth more than money.
    Spend them wisely.

334. No snowflake in an avalanche ever feels responsible.

335. Do onto others as you wish others do onto you.

336. Opportunities surround you if you know where to look.

337. Soon life will become more interesting.

338. Peace comes from within. Seek it from yourself.

339. Your body and mind can only take you so far. Your spirit will lead you to your destiny.

340. The individual threads you spin are part of the greater design that serves us all.

341. One who is too insistent on his own views, finds few to agree with him.

342. It's not the years in your life, but the life
in your years that counts.

343. Compassion is a way of being.

344. Behavior defines you more than your beliefs.

345. Work is either fun or drudgery. It depends on your attitude.

346. New people will bring you new realizations, especially big issues.

347. The human body was designed to walk, run or stop; it wasn't built for coasting.

348. No need to worry! You will always have everything that you need.

349. Only you can decide what is important to you.

350. Sever the ignorant doubt in your heart with the sword of self-knowledge.

351. Determination will get you through this.

352. It is a great piece of skill to know how to guide your luck. Even while waiting for it.

353. What is contained in everything? Wisdom.

354. Sometime advice is what we ask for when we already know the answer.

355. Enjoy life. This is not a dress rehearsal.

356. Courtesy begins in the home.

357. Obstacles are frightful things you see when you take your eyes off the goal.

358. It's not the end. Stay with it.

359. It is the most gratifying goal that must begin with a small achievement.

360. Relish the transitions in your life. They will happen regardless.

361. The life you live must be the one
you chose and make.

362. You will be successful
in love.

363. Nothing in life is to be feared.
It is only to be understood.

364. Don't find fault,
find a remedy.

365. No man is a failure who
is enjoying life.

366. The harder the fall, the higher the
bounce.

367. Poverty is no disgrace.

368. Life is full of wonders... explore
what's around you.

369. May you grow rich.

370. Only the person who risks is truly free.

371. Despair is criminal...a crime against yourself.

372. Failure is the chance to do better next time.

373. Don't get so caught up in the daily grind that you never find time to enjoy yourself.

374. Examine the situation before you act impulsively.

375. You must know how the system works before you can change it.

376. Never confuse a single defeat with a final defeat.

377. He who expects no gratitude shall never be disappointed.

378. Thinking is the soul talking to its self.

379. Only the dead have seen the end of war.

380. Give a book, you give the possibility of a new life.

381. A greedy man is always in need.

382. To be loved, one must be loveable.

383. Knowing your opponent's intentions, gives you strategic knowledge.

384. Love is a warm fire to keep the soul warm.

385. Compassion will cure more than condemnation.

386. Do not step on anyone on the way to the top.

387. Courage is grace under pressure.

388. Early to bed and early to rise makes a person healthy, wealthy, and wise.

389. Joy shared is doubled. Sorrow shared is halved.

390. Dogs have owners; cats staffs.

391. Everything originates from the seed of determination.

392. Experience is the name everyone gives to their mistakes.

393. Soon you will be sitting on top of the world.

394. In great attempts it is glorious even to fail.

395. Joy is the feeling of grinning on the inside.

396. Your diamonds are in your backyard.
Just dig to find them.

397. Before you roar, please take a deep breath.

398. Care and attention to the key relationships in your life will pay off.

399. Example is better than perception.

400. Faith is knowing there is an ocean when you can only see the stream.

401. Be smart, be intelligent, and be informed.

402. Keep your feet on the ground and your thoughts at lofty heights.

403. Conquer your fears. Otherwise, your fears will conquer you.

404. Don't be afraid to take a big step. You can't cross a chasm in two small jumps.

405. It is always darkest before dawn.

406. Many people who have power become a deaf-mute.

407. Before you can do something you must first be something.

408. Do what is right, not what you should.

409. To find yourself, you must leave the city of comfort and follow our intuition.

410. Establish harmony and balance in your life.

411. Enthusiastic leadership gets you a promotion when you least expect it.

412. I hear and I forget. I see and I remember.

413. One who does nothing but wait for his ship to come has already missed the boat.

414. Life is too short to waste time hating anyone.

415. Everywhere you choose to go, friendly faces will greet you.

416. Do not hesitate to look for help. An extra hand should always be welcomed.

417. Excuses are easy to manufacture and hard to sell.

418. If you love something, set it free…if it returns, keep it and love it forever.

419. Every truly great accomplishment is at first impossible.

420. Careful thinking will command respect.

421. Broke is only temporary;
poor is a state of mind.

422. Gratitude is not only the greatest
of virtues, but the parent of all
others.

423. Everyone has a photographic
memory. Some just don't have
film.

424. If your desires are not extravagant
they will be granted.

425. Fear and desire – two sides
of the same coin.

426. It's a good thing that life is not as
serious as it seems to the waiter.

427. Take the initiative and others will
support you

428. Be willing to give an extra effort that separates you from second place.

429. You have to tolerate the rain to find your rainbow,

430. Get to the point and keep it clear and simple.

431. Even a small gift could mean so much to someone today.

432. Seize every second of your life and savor it.

433. It a turtle doesn't have a shell, is it naked or homeless?

434. Happy event will take place shortly in your home.

435. Correction does much, but encouragement everything.

436. Lies and sorrow may float through the air, but truth and happiness live inside you.

437. Luck sometimes visits a fool, but it never sits down with him.

438. Engage in group activities that further transformation.

439. It's not what you know but what you USE of what you know that counts.

440. Learn to listen, not just hear.

441. Do not give a fish to a hungry man; teach him how to fish.

442. Man is born to live but

not prepared to live.

443.   Demonstrate refinement in
       everything you do.

444.   Love is a present you can give
       every single day you live.

445.   Enjoy what you have, hope for
       what you lack.

446.   It is better to deal with problems
       before they arise.

447.   Cleaning up the Past will always
       clear up the Future.

448.   Don't let your limitations
       overshadow your talents.

449.   Cut through organizational
       impediments and get
       some real work done.

450. Life is an active verb.

451. Spend more time looking where you're going, not where you've been.

452. Domestic conditions demand your attention.

453. Do it because you love it.

454. Better aim at the moon than shoot into a well.

455. If you never change your mind, why have one?

456. Dream lofty dreams, and as you dream, so shall you become.

457. One's fear of dying robs one of Life's greatness.

458.   Don't ignore minor detail; they are
       the key to your success.

459.   Don't take life too seriously; laugh
       and smile at it once in a while.

460.   Collect your thoughts and act
       accordingly.

461.   Don't be pushed by your
       problems. Be led by your dreams.

462.   It's is very possible that you will
       achieve greatness in your lifetime.

463.   Do you want to be a power in the
       world? Then be yourself.

464.   Even a broken clock is right
       two times a day.

465. Emptiness is the mother of all things.

466. Don't be fooled by first impressions.

467. Happiness is not a reward, it's a consequence.

468. Moderate your appetite so that with a little you may be content.

469. Any job, big or small; do it right, or not at all.

470. Do not demand for one's soul if you already got his heart.

471. Be demonstrative, but do it with dignity.

472. Things are turning for the bright side.

473. Be willing to give the extra effort that separates the winner from others.

474. Courage is rightly considered the foremost of the virtues, as all others depend upon it.

475. Devotion will make you feel more complete.

476. Calamity is the touchstone of a brave mind.

477. Be happy with the person you are. Don't let anyone tell you otherwise.

478. Choosing what you want to do, and when to do it, is an act of creation.

479. Those who judge only by first
impressions are
oft times fools.

480. It takes courage to grow up and
turn out to be
who you really are.

481. He who talks but does not speak is
mute.

482. Courtesy cost nothing.

483. There's nothing more dangerous
than an idea if it's the only one
you have.

484. Although it feels like a roller
coaster now, life will calm down.

485. Those who do not remember the
past are condemned
to repeat it.

486. Do what you can with what you have, where you are.

487. Courtesy is one habit that never goes out of style.

488. Don't be fooled by first impressions.

489. To beautify externally is like a glass rose; one false move and it can crack.

490. You are the jailer of your potential. Use the key to set it free!

491. Delay is the antidote for anger.

492. There are no rules…and they just changed!

493. The beginning and the ending are the same point in time.

494. Do the right thing because it is the right to do.

495. Discipline is wisdom and vice versa.

496. Depend on the predictability and steadiness of life to support you.

497. Listening well is as essential to all true conversation as speaking well.

498. Affirm it, visualize it, believe it, and it will actualize itself.

499. Everyone has someone to love.

500. Change is inevitable, except for vending machines.

501. Be on the alert for new opportunities.

502. Begin…the rest is easy.

503. Consume less. Share more. Enjoy life.

504. Cookies go stale. Fortunes are forever.

505. Try not to stand on your own side during an argument.

506. From now on your kindness will lead you to success.

507. Three can keep a secret, if you get rid of two.

508. Be careful or you could fall for some tricks today.

509. Believe in your abilities, confidence will lead you on.

510. Compromise is always wrong if it means sacrificing a principle.

511. Love is the first feeling people feel,
because love is nice.

512. Don't be over confident with first impression of others.

513. Holding on is best way to lose out.

514. Expect a change for the better in your job or status in the future.

515. Difficulty at the beginning usually means ease at the end.

516. Vacation can wait. Stick to the project till the end.

517. It is not where you stand in this world, but the direction you are moving.

518. Circumstances do not make the man, they merely reveal himself to himself.

519. It's not having, it's getting.

520. He who knows he has enough is rich.

521. Do not let ambitions overshadow small successes.

522. Mutual assistance in despair will make the ugly situation be fairer.

523. It's not the will to win, but the will to prepare to win that makes a difference.

524. By working hard, you get to play hard…guilt-free.

525. Courtesy is one habit that never goes out of style.

526. Many successes will accompany you this year.

527. Courtesy is one of the best peacemakers.

528. Courage conquers all things; it even gives strength to the body.

529. Fortitude is the guard and support of the other virtues.

530. Dream lofty dreams, and as you dream, so shall you become.

531. He who hears but not Listens, is deaf.

532. To be eighty years young is more cheerful than being forty years old.

533. If you look in the right places, you can find some good offerings.

534. Look around; happiness is trying to catch you.

535. The seeds of payback are sown daily.

536. To think is easy; to act is difficult. To act as one thinks is the most difficult of all.

537. In this world it is not what we take
up, but what we give up,
  that makes us rich.

538. It is always darkest before dawn.

539. Even the toughest of days have
bright spots, just do your best.

540. Don't take life too seriously,
  laugh and smile at it
  once in a while.

541. Having more money does not
insure happiness.

542. A chance meeting opens new
doors to success and friendship.

543. Blessed is that man whose passion
is his work.

544. Every action has a counter action,
even if you see it

or not.

545. There is absolutely no substitute
for
a genuine lack of preparation.

546. Set your goals high and you will
always move forward.

547. Enjoy life! It is better to be happy
than wise.

548. Minds are like parachutes. They
only function when they are open.

549. Believe it can be done.

550. An ounce of care is worth
a pound of cure.

551. Man has a limitless capacity to
achieve goodness.

552. It's time you asked that special someone out
on a date.

553. Your hearing will improve the quieter you become.

554. It is a silly fish that is caught twice with the same bait.

555. Land is always in the mind of the flying bird.

556. A man without aim is like a clock without hands,
useless if it turns or if it stands still.

557. A very attractive person has a message for you.

558. There is just one life for each of us; our own.

559. Commitment is the daily triumph of integrity over skepticism.

560. Action speaks nothing, without the Motive.

561. Fate loves the fearless.

562. Change is constant. How it's handled determines future.

563. We don't know who we are until we see what we can do.

564. Take time to deliberate; but when the time for action arrives, stop thinking and act.

565. The most important thing is to never stop questioning.

566. Expect much of yourself and little of others.

567. You must look at yourself through
your soul's eyes to see the beauty
of your
own being.

568. Forgive the action,
forget the intent.

569. A good memory is fine but the
ability to forget is the one true test
of greatness.

570. Dance like no one is watching.

571. When all you have is a hammer,
everything looks like a nail.

572. A short saying oft contains
much wisdom.

573. There is one cause of human failure. That is man's lack of faith in his true self.

574. Time to break out of that corner, unstuck that rut.

575. We don't have to change friends if we understand that friends change.

576. We are taught by every person we meet.

577. Always accept yourself the way you are at the moment.

578. Be smart, but never show it.

579. Ask advice, but use your own common sense.

580. He who loves a project is the least qualified to judge its value to others.

581. Tomorrow morning, take a left turn as soon as you leave home.

582. Fresh ideas are not always the best ideas.

583. Failure is opportunity in disguise.

584. He who waits to do a great deal of good all at once, will never do anything.

585. Think of how you can assist on a problem, not who to blame for the problem.

586. To love and beloved are blessings.

587. We must not become complacent over any success.

588. Ulcers are caused not so much by what we eat as what's eating us.

589. Generosity will repay itself sooner than you imagine.

590. To affirm is to make firm.
591. There is no glory unless you put yourself on the line.

592. Things are turning for the bright side.

593. Action speaks nothing, without the Motive.

594. After readying every emotion, there is understanding entering the realm.

595. What is to give light must endure the burning.

596. A perfect statue never comes from a bad mould.

597. A bargain is not a bargain unless you can use the product.

598. Thorough preparation makes its own luck.

599. Courage is the form of every virtue at the testing point.

600. Fear not, worry not.

601. There's more to balance than not falling over.

602. Attitudes are the forerunners of conditions.

603. To be a success in business,

be daring, be first,
be different.

604. It's all right to have butterflies in your stomach. Just get them to fly in formation.

605. Believe in yourself and you will succeed.

606. To have a fighting chance one must have a fighting spirit.

607. An hour with friends is worth more than ten with strangers.

608. Everything that we see is a shadow cast by that which we do not see.

609. Dispel negativity through creative activities.

610. Time heals most everything.

Give it time.

611. All troubles you have can pass
     away very quickly.

612. We all have a lot more in common
     than it seems.

613. A good way to keep healthy is
     to eat more Chinese food.

614. Don't be afraid to smile, you never
     know who's falling in love with it!

615. There is a true and sincere
     friendship between you both.

616. Broke is only temporary; poor is a
     state of mind that you can change
     with thought.

617. Want to catch the fishes, one must
     go home to build

the net first.

618. Trust your intuition. The universe is guiding your life.

619. Tonight will be a lucky night.

620. Question: What is K.M.S.?
Answer: Keep Mouth Shut,
the golden rule.

621. It is where you go and what you do when you get there that will speak who you are.

622. A single kind word will keep one warm for years.

623. Calamity is the touchstone of a brave mind.

624. Act well your part; there honor lies.

625. The time is right to make good friends.

626. All personal breakthroughs begin with a change in beliefs.

627. Ability is not something to be shown off.

628. Develop an appreciation for the present moment.

629. The future is the most expensive luxury in the world.

630. All the effort you are making will ultimately pay off.

631. What is temporary has to be temporary. Just don't let it last longer than a year.

632. What you will discover will be yourself.

633. Character is much easier kept than recovered.

634. 42.7 percent of all statistics are made up on the spot.

635. There's a good chance of a romantic encounter soon.

636. The finest eloquence is that which gets things done.

637. We treat this world of ours as though we had a spare in the trunk.

638. There is no mistake so great as that of being always right.

639. Be on the alert to recognize your prime at whatever time it may occur.

640. An investment in knowledge always pays the best interest.

641. All the news you receive will be positive and uplifting.

642. This is not a day to take risks. Diplomacy rules today.

643. It is never a shame to learn from others.

644. What is not started will never get finished.

645. A friend asks only for your time, not your money.

646. Faith is the bird that feels the light and sings while the dawn is still dark.

647. Those that love rumors hate a peaceful life.

648. That which is painful to the body may be profitable to the soul.

649. It is not the outside riches but the inside ones that produce happiness.

650. There is no reference for beauty.

651. Treasure your good memories and you need not worry about ending a banquet.

652. There is no fear for the one who's thought is not confused.

653. Executive ability is prominent in your makeup.

654. Utility is when you have plumbing; luxury is when you have a pool.

655. We will not know the worth of water until the well is dry.

656. There are no shortcuts to any place worth going.

657. Treasure what you have.

658. Be receptive to new ideas from all fronts.

659. Most people are graduates of The School of Hard Knocks. Where did you graduate?

660. There is no time like the pleasant.

661. May life throw you a pleasant
     curve.

662. You cannot use the same thinking
     that created the problem to solve it.

663. Never does nature say one thing
     and wisdom another.

664. Alter ideas and you alter the world.

665. Morality is truth in bloom.

666. In this world of contradiction,
     it's better to be
     merry than wise.

667. The care and sensitivity you show
     towards others will return to you.

668. Have faith in the force of right and
     not in the right of force.

669. Answer what your heart prompts you.

670. The years teach much which the days never know.

671. Today is a huge improvement over yesterday.

672. Be on the alert for new opportunities.

673. Luck will visit you on the next new moon.

674. Do what is right, not what you should.

675. A small gift can bring joy to the whole family.

676. We cannot direct the wind but we can adjust the sails

677. Make sure to laugh everyday…it's good for your health.

678. Take time to relax when you don't have time for it.

679. Make your life an exclamation not an explanation.

680. Excellence is the difference between what you do and what you are capable of doing.

681. To be mature is to accept imperfections.

682. Life begins just beyond the border of your comfort zone.

683. A beautiful person is with you, confide your problems.

684. Be not afraid of growing slowly,
be afraid of remaining standing
still.

685. To see an old friend is as agreeable
as a good meal.

686. The issue isn't what you're saying;
mostly it's the way.

687. Your character is
your destiny.

688. A smile is nearly always inspired
by another smile.

689. Don't expect to find one right way
to make yourself more creative.

690. The first step toward change is
awareness. The second step is
acceptance.

691. Any impatience you show will only create more stress.

692. Many new friends will be attracted to your friendly, charming ways.

693. We must have old memories and young hopes.

694. An investment in yourself will pay dividends for the rest of your life.

695. Every job is a self-portrait of the person who did it.

696. Autograph your work with excellence.

697. Giving will make you smile.

698. To know the universe you first must know yourself.

699. A danger foreseen is half avoided.

700. There is no greater pleasure than seeing your loved ones prosper.

701. Don't waste time on what might have been.

702. There are two ways to shine. Be the candle or, the mirror that reflects it.

703. Treat yourself with the same dignity and respect you give others.

704. Do not fear failure for it lights the pathway to success.

705. Humor is best weapon against sarcasm. Laugh at it.

706. Three things cannot be long hidden: The Sun, the Moon, and the Truth.

707. The speed of the leader determines the rate of the pack.

708. Those who walk in other's tracks leave no footprints.

709. Focus your attention.

710. Many possibilities are available to you. Work a little harder to earn them.

711. The road to success is often a lonely one.

712. Avert misunderstandings by calm, poise and balance.

713. The impossible is only what others think you can't achieve.

714. Failure is a greater teacher
     than success.

715. Balance your life with
     a little sweet and sour.

716. Adversity is the first path to truth.

717. What we acquire without sweat we
     give away
     without regret.

718. An optimistic attitude is half of
     success.

719. A small donation is called for.
     It's the right thing to do.

720. There is no such thing as
     an ordinary cat.

721. The small courtesies sweeten life,
     greater ones ennoble it.

722. There is no sorrow in the world
that a long hot bath wouldn't help.

723. Teach oneself : explore
the old and deduce the new.

724. Be on the alert to recognize your
prime at whatever time of your life
it may occur.

725. It is by those who have suffered
that the world is most advanced.

726. Time heals all wounds.

727. We judge others by actions;
we judge ourselves by our
intentions.

728. A new environment makes all the
difference in the world.

729. Absence sharpens love, but presence strengthens it.

730. A person is not wise simply because one talks a lot.

731. A romantic evening awaits you tonight.

732. To courageously shoulder the responsibility of one's mistake is character.

733. The answer will not come to you; you need to look for it.

734. People are as happy as they make up their minds to be.

735. In the end, all things will be known.

736. A man can fail many times, but he isn't a failure until he gives up.

737. A dose of adversity is often as needful as a dose of medicine.

738. There is but one cause of human failure; that is man's lack of faith in his true self.

739. Experience is reflective, like a still pool.

740. Time is not measured by a watch but by moments.

741. Maintaining takes less energy than attaining.

742. Any idea seriously entertained tends to bring about the realization of itself.

743. We grow great by dreams. All big men are dreamers.

744. There is no greater gift than good health. Cherish it always.

745. Courtesy is a business asset
— a gain, never a loss.

746. Truth can be harsh, but it can helpful.

747. Aim for the sky, because even if you miss, you'll still be among the stars.

748. Truth is an unpopular subject, as it is unquestionably correct.

749. To rule with virtue is like the North Star has its place
in the sky.

750. Take a vacation, you will have unexpected gains.

751. You are the harvest of your past plantings.

752. Many possibilities are open to you
– work a little harder.

753. Greatest fool of all is the man who
fools himself.

754. Your greatest fortune is the friends
and family you have.

755. A close friend reveals a hidden
talent.

756. No problem leaves you where you
found it.

757. Your happiness is before you, not
behind! Cherish it.

758. A billionaire's joke is always
funny.

759. This is your time for love and
affection.

760. Your greatest fortune is the friends and family you have.

761. Think of how you can assist on a problem... not who to blame.

762. Bread today is better than cake tomorrow.

763. Compassion is a way of being.

764. Leadership is action, not position.

765. A day without smiling is a day wasted.

766. Listening, not imitation, may be the sincerest form of flattery.

767. Devotion will make you feel more complete.

768. The wisest owl hears all before he flies.

769. To be able to look back upon one's past life with satisfaction is to live twice.

770. You will reach the highest possible point in your business or profession.

771. A journey of a thousand miles must begin with a single step.

772. A modest man never talks to himself.

773. Determination is the wake-up call to the human will.

774. You are your God's gift to you; what you do with it is your gift to your God.

775. To know oneself, one should assert oneself.

776. The joyful energy of the day
     will have a positive
       effect on you.

777. There is no greater cure for misery than hard work.

778. Trust is earned by many deeds.
     And can be lost with one miss
     deed.

779. Only tears can bring the dreamer back to earth.

780. Success is to believe in yourself.

781. Failing to prepare is preparing to fail.

782. The simplest answer is to act.

783. You are going to have a comfortable old age.

784. This instant is the only time there is.

785. Value your present moments.

786. Success comes in cans, not in cannots.

787. Happier days are ahead for you. Struggle has ended.

788. Suppose you can get what you want, what would you have to give up?

789. Lack of compassion is as rude as too many tears.

790. Stand tall! Don't look down upon yourself.

791. Character matters; leadership descends from character.

792. Someone from your past has returned to steal your heart.

793. Search your own heart with all diligence for out of it flows the issues of life

794. The one you love is closer than you think.

795. This is not a day to take risks. Diplomacy rules today.

796. The mighty oak was once a little nut that stood its ground.

797. Don't forget, you are always on our minds.

798. Physical activity will dramatically improve
   your outlook today.

799. A warm smile is testimony of
   a generous nature.

800. A secret admirer will soon
   send you a sign of affection.

801. Love asks you no questions, and
   gives you endless support.

802. Love always and deeply.

803. He who throws dirt is losing
   ground.

804. In the end there are three things
   that last: faith, hope and love.

805. Love is for the lucky and the
   brave.

806. If you continually give, you will
continually have.

807. If you would be loved, love
and be lovable.

808. Your heart will always make itself
known through your words.

809. Do not mistake temptation for
opportunity.

810. We can only do small things
with great love.

811. Love is like wildflowers...it is
often found in unlikely places.

812. Love is the only medicine
for a broken heart.

813. You can always find happiness at
work on Friday.

814. A woman who seeks to be equal with men lacks ambition.

815. Change is the constant in life.

816. The greatest danger could be your stupidity.

817. Plan for many pleasures.

818. He who laughs at himself never runs out of things to laugh at.

819. He who laughs last is laughing at you.

820. A closed mouth gathers no feet.

821. A conclusion is simply the place where you got tired of thinking.

822. You find beauty in ordinary things; do not lose this ability.

823. A cynic is only a frustrated optimist.

824. Something you lost will turn up soon.

825. Ideas are like children, there are none so wonderful as your own.

826. It takes more than good memory to have good memories.

827. A thrilling time is in your immediate future.

828. Your blessing is no more than being safe and sound for a lifetime.

829. Your joyfulness of life prolongs your days.

830. Your heart is pure, your mind clear, and your soul devout.

831. Excitement and intrigue follow you wherever you go.

832. A pleasant surprise is in store for you.

833. As the purse is emptied the heart is filled.

834. Be mischievous and you not be lonesome.

835. You have a deep appreciation of the arts and music.

836. Your flair for being creative takes
an important place in your life.

837. Don't forget you are always
on our minds.

838. Your artistic talents win the
approval and applause of others.

839. Pray for what you want,
but work for what you need.

840. Your hidden talents become
obvious to those around you.

841. Your greatest fortune is
your large number of friends.

842. A firm friendship will prove the
foundation of your success in life.

843. Don't ask. Don't say. Everything lies in silence.

844. Look for new outlets for your own creative abilities.

845. Prepare to accept a wondrous opportunity ahead.

846. There are no rules, and they have all changed.

847. Fame, riches and romance are yours for the asking.

848. Good luck is the result of good planning.

849. Good things are being said about you.

850. Smiling often can make you look and feel younger.

851. People speak well of you.

852. Fear is excitement in need of
an attitude adjustment.

853. Your life will be happy and
peaceful.

854. A friend is a present you give
yourself.

855. A family member will soon do
something that will make you
proud.

856. A quiet evening with friends is the
best tonic for a bad day.

857. A single kind word will keep one
warm for years.

858. Anger begins with folly,
and ends with regret.

859. Generosity and perfection are your everlasting goals.

860. Happy news is
on its way to you.

861. If your desires are not extravagant they will be granted.

862. Let there be magic in your smile and firmness in your handshake.

863. Nature, Time and Patience
are the three best physicians.

864. Strong and bitter words indicate a weak cause.

865. You will have a very pleasant experience.

866. Your everlasting Patience will be rewarded sooner or later.

867. Make two grins grow where
there was only one grouch before.

868. You will step on the soil of many
countries.

869. The privilege of a lifetime is being
who you are.

870. You will take a chance on
something in the near future.

871. Don't be afraid to reach out to
make new friends.

872. Love is the triumph of imagination
over intelligence.

873. Wanting to be like someone else is
Envy. Accepting one's self brings
happiness.

874. Much more grows in the garden
than that planted there.

875. One who admires you greatly is hidden before your eyes.

876. Only love lets us see normal things as extraordinary.

877. The greatest gift is love.

878. This is no limit to love's trust nor its power to endure.

879. Those who have love, have wealth beyond measure.

880. If the road of life was straight, without bumps and turns, life would be boring.

881. Winning one's heart must be earned, not given as gift.

882. Your heart is a place to draw true happiness.

883. Your true blessings are those whom you love.

884. Marriage is not a mad dash to the altar; it is a marathon of living.

885. Your heart is a place to draw true happiness.

886. Knowledge of your path can not be substituted by following your path.

887. Your everlasting patience will be rewarded sooner…or later.

888. Your great attention to detail is both a blessing and a curse.

889. Your ability to juggle many tasks will take you far.

890. A friend asks only for your time, not your money.

891. You will be invited to an exciting event.

892. Choice, whether right or wrong, is the divine teacher.

893. Reality of time only exists with you.

894. Reaching the mountain top is the beginning point of your climb.

895. All events are given to you from which you learn.

896. Know your limits so you

can smash them to reach
magnificence.

897. Our first and last love
is self love.

898. None of the secrets of success
work unless you do.

899. An open mind is like a window, it
lets in fresh air.

900. If you only follow others' paths,
you will never find your own.

901. Today is a lucky day for one who
is cheerful and optimistic.

902. You were born with the skill to
communicate with people easily.

903. Listen to what other people say, not hear only what you want to hear.

904. Acceptance of who you are grants you the chance to change.

905. To find your soul. You must first find the joys of life.

906. Self is not something you find, but what you create.

907. Every flower is a soul blooming. What kind of flower are you?

908. Readiness must be converted to willingness to find your role in the Universe.

909. The end of your exploring will lead to when you began.

910. Your "Promised Land" always lies on the other side of the wilderness.

911. If you are afraid of dying, you will never truly live.

912. The greatest cause of deafness is a closed mind.

913. You can't experience the world living under a mushroom.

914. Your journey is more important than your destination.

915. Plan to live forever; live like you will die tomorrow.

916. Life without passion is like egg fu young without eggs.

917. For most people chopsticks help you burn calories while you eat.

918. Desire without execution leads to disappointment.

919. One who strives for the best rarely comes up with a hand full of mud.

920. Saving for the future will pad your retirement bed.

921. Teas are like people. Many varieties. All interesting. Imbibe.

922. Your success will be driven by desire, fueled by commitment.

923. Heaven and Hell are within you. You determine your residence.

924. Take action now on those things you value the most.

925. The best gift one can give
     is a good example.

926. The best things in life are not free,
     they're earned.

927. If you just tiptoe through the tulips
     you will miss the essence and
     fragrance of the journey.

928. Marriage is accepting the faults of
     your other for the betterment of the
     relationship.

929. A roadblock directs one to a better
     way to proceed.

930. Your path to success will be a
     meandering one.

931. The smart person surrounds them
     self with smarter people.

932. Very few horses lead races from start to finish. They follow, then move to lead.

933. Most times animals are better judge of people than people.

934. Your retirement account and a beggar's bowl have much in common.

935. You reach out for success, but keep your feet on the ground.

936. You find people exciting.

937. The more you are engaged with the world the more tolerant you are of it.

938. Your road to success will have many twists, turns and detours.

939. You are reserve and that is why people listen when you speak.

940. Competition reduces many thoughts of reality to one reality.

941. You help others to change by not attempting to change them.

942. Intention without determination is an idling car.

943. When everyday is like everyday, it is time to change your way.

944. Your ability to remain objective in a crisis drives others crazy.

945. You see what can be, not just what is there, or not there.

946. Do not be embarrassed to reach out to others for assistance.

947. Grow as tall as you can, keeping your feet on the ground.

948. A good book and a quiet evening, can be better than a night of partying.

949. Happiness is liking who you are, not just what you have.

950. The number of true friends can be counted on one's hand.

951. Life is a relay, one generation handing off its knowledge to the next generation.

952. When exercising, stretch your mind as well as your body.

953. A mind set in concrete is subject to breakage.

954. You are a person who loves the company of others.

955. Healthy living requires nurturing the mind as well as the body.

956. Running from one's problems usually ends up with one colliding into the wall of reality.

957. Only sing the self-pity song in the shower.

958. Life is like a budding flower, you must let it unfold at its own pace or risk destroying it.

959. Prejudice and fear are weeds to be pruned from one's Garden of Life.

960. Perfection is only a panicle you can fall from.

961. The wise person does not mistake cunning for stupidity.

962. You motivate people to do better through your own actions.

963. Your thoughts will continue to influence people long after you have departed.

964. Seek the truth as the person whose hair is on fire seeks a lake.

965. Desire without urgency rarely leads to less than desirable results.

966. Know the difference between a friend and an acquaintance.

967. It takes a husband many years to realize his wife has always been in charge.

968. You carry your greatest fortune within you.

969. The person who sticks his toe in Life's river cannot know the exhilaration of total emersion.

970. You move easily among different groups of people.

971. Reserve your wisdom for those who have ears that listen.

972. You are the type of person who listens first and speaks second.

973. Your fortune is what you make of your life.

974. Embrace Change. It's not an Adversary. It's Opportunity!

975. The opposite of Love is not Hate, but indifference.

976. Life's challenge is to Survive, Strive, and then Thrive.

977. Your reward will far outweigh your effort to achieve it.

978. Face facts with dignity.

979. Ambition makes the world go round.

980. Speak when you have something worthwhile to say;
     then, people will listen.

981. Look before you leap, but hesitate and you're lost.

982. You base your decisions on facts, not hearsay, rumor or innuendo.

983. Get out of your work shell and explore the beautiful world around you.

984. Something free is rarely appreciated for its true worth.

985. You see the obvious where others see nothing.

986. Those who speak the loudest have little comprehension of their subject.

987. Ignorance is the greatest roadblock to understanding.

988. You must not just listen, you must think before stating your view.

989. Dare to live the life you want.

990. Don't let life kill your life's dream.

991. A foot. A device for finding furniture in the dark.

992. The world has always been a mess. It is your job to find your place in it.

993. No one has a good enough memory to make a   successful liar.

994. People say you have sharp sense ad superb intellect.

995. Faithless is he who quits when the road darkens.

996. Release your inner love of life so that more people can see you for the great person you truly are.

997. Failure is only the opportunity to begin more intelligently.

998. Financial hardship in your life is coming to an end!

999. The beginning will lead you to the end which will be the beginning.

1000. Relationships are like fingers of your hand. "One" cannot do much.

1001. Everything will work out for the best in the end.

THANK YOU

I hope you have enjoyed this collection of wise, witty, wacky and whimsical sayings as much as I have had in finding and assembling them. Now here are a few more tidbits of information.

****

A BIT (OR SHOULD IT BE A BITE) OF HISTORY

The Chinese Fortune cookie, like chop suey, is not Chinese but an American invention. And, in fact it may have originated with the Japanese population that immigrated to the United States The exact provenance of fortune cookies is unclear, though various immigrant groups in California claim to have popularized them in the early 20th century, basing their recipe on a traditional Japanese cracker. Fortune cookies have been summarized as being introduced by the Japanese, popularized by the Chinese, but ultimately ... consumed by Americans.

Chinese or Japanese, Angelino or San Franciscan?

One history of the fortune cookie claims that David Jung, a Chinese immigrant living in

Los Angeles and founder of the Hong Kong Noodle Company, invented the cookie in 1918. Concerned about the poor he saw wandering near his shop, he created the cookie and passed them out free on the streets. Each cookie contained a strip of paper with an inspirational Bible scripture on it, written for Jung by a Presbyterian minister.

Another history claims that the fortune cookie was invented in San Francisco by a Japanese immigrant named Makoto Hagiwara. Hagiwara was a gardener who designed the famous Japanese Tea Garden in Golden Gate Park. An anti-Japanese mayor fired him from his job around the turn of the century, but later a new mayor reinstated him.

Grateful to those who had stood by him during his period of hardship, Hagiwara created a cookie in 1914 that included a thank you note inside. He passed them out at the Japanese Tea Garden, and began serving them there regularly. In 1915, they were displayed at the Panama-Pacific Exhibition, San Francisco's world fair.

Judicial Activism

In 1983, San Francisco's pseudo-legal Court of Historical Review held a mock trial to determine the origins of the fortune cookie. (In the past, the Court had ruled on such pressing topics as the veracity of Mark Twain's quote, "The coldest winter I ever spent was a summer in San Francisco" and the origins of the Martini.)

To no one's surprise, the judge (a real-life federal judge from San Francisco) ruled in favor of San Francisco. Included among the evidence was a fortune cookie whose message read: "S.F. Judge who rules for L.A. Not Very Smart Cookie." Equally unsurprising, Los Angeles denounced the ruling.

From Confucius to Smiley Faces

Fortune cookies became common in Chinese restaurants after World War II. Desserts were not traditionally part of Chinese cuisine; thus the funny shaped cookies offered Americans something familiar with an exotic flair.

Although there have been a few cases reported of individuals actually *liking* the texture and flavor of fortune cookies, most consider the fortune to be the essence of the cookie. Early fortunes featured Biblical sayings, or aphorisms from Confucius, Aesop, or Ben Franklin.

Later, fortunes included jokes, recommended lottery numbers, smiley faces, and sage, if hackneyed, advice. Politicians have used them in campaigns, and fortunes have been customized for weddings and birthday parties.

Today messages are variously cryptic, nonsensical, feel-good, hectoring, bland, or mystifying. In essence, you can now have your fortune "as you like it."

From Chopsticks to High Tech
Fortune cookies were originally made by hand using chopsticks. In 1964, Edward Louie of San Francisco's Lotus Fortune Cookie Company, automated the process by creating a machine that folds the dough and slips in the fortune. Today, the world's largest fortune cookie manufacturer, Wonton Food Inc. of Long Island City, Queens ships out 60 million cookies a month.

Makers of Chinese Fortune Cookies

There are approximately 3 billion fortune cookies made each year around the world, the vast majority of them are consumed n in the United States.

The largest manufacturer is Wonton Food Inc., headquartered in New York. It makes over 4.5 million fortune cookies per day.

Other large manufacturers are:
Baily International in the Midwest and Peking Noodle in the Los Angeles area. Tsue Chong Co. in Seattle, WA.

In closing, please remember:

The Past is a Memory.
The Future is a Dream.
Only the Present is Real...
It's The Now.
Live and Enjoy the Moment...
Every Moment!
Because,
who knows what's next.